TO HELL AND BACK

By Ann Denise Parsons

'One Million People Commit Suicide Every Year'
The World Health Organization

All rights reserved, no part of this publication may be reproduced by any means, electronic, mechanical, or photocopying, documentary, film, or otherwise without prior permission of the publisher.

>Published by:
>Chipmunkapublishing
>PO Box 6872
>Brentwood
>Essex
>CM13 1ZT
>United Kingdom
>
>http://www.chipmunkapublishing.com

Copyright © 2007 Ann Denise Parsons

TO HELL AND BACK

A SHORT STORY OF MY LIFE

BY ANN DENISE PARSONS

Firstly, I was aware from when I was a teenager that my dad had something 'wrong' with him. Later I was to find out that it was because he was an alcoholic. I first became aware of Alateen (12 step fellowship for teenagers of alcoholics) when I was 16 and went to my first meeting in Chelsea shortly afterwards, I then drove to Enfield when I was 17 (having passed my driving test first time at this age) to attend Alateen, where it was started by two American's – Bonny and George. These meetings were great and gave me the chance to talk about stuff that I couldn't really talk to anyone else about.

I was always out at disco's especially Epping Forest Country Club and the West End and had loads of friends and boyfriends. I also had a horse that my parents bought me when I was 16, mostly though it was my mother who persuaded my dad eventually. I kept my horse for 5 years and used to love riding in Epping Forest, I also did show-jumping and cross-country eventing on her and used to have great fun and won plenty of rosettes. My sister also was bought a horse and we used to go out riding together, we also had two cats, a Labrador dog and lived in a very expensive area of Loughton in Essex in a huge detached five bedroomed house overlooking the countryside of Ongar and Abridge, (we also had a gardener and a cleaner). We lived close to Epping Forest and I had grown up in Loughton since I was five years of age and lived a very comfortable privileged life, apart from the times with my father being an alcoholic and his irrational behaviour which got progressively worse as time went by. He was lucky that in the business he had, which employed about thirty people he had very competent managers who virtually ran the business for him when he was in the pub drinking all day.

I broke up with a serious relationship, which lasted for five years, at the age of 21, my mother pointed me in the direction of a counsellor (who was also a vicar) who lived in Orpington in Kent, I was so upset I agreed to go. (From what I have now found out about the whole mess at this time, was that my parents were seeing this particular 'vicar' for counselling too, which to me made sense years later as to why this vicar was presurising me to leave home, as he knew from talking to my parents that things were not as they seemed at home, we later found out that about this time my dad was having an affair with a girl at work who was the same age as me then (which was 21) and was also married (I saw them together on a couple occasions whilst driving but thought it was work related), also over the years I have found out that a counsellor should never see anyone from the same family unless it is family therapy as this is not good practice and 'unethical').

This vicar talked to me about leaving home and in particular going to work on a kibbutz in Israel, so that's what I did. I gave up a promising career as a shorthand secretary to three directors, and at the age of 21 left home for the first time and went to Israel. I ended up on the Lebanese Border, it was a nerve racking situation because of the war that was going on in 1982 when Israel was fighting in Lebanon, and I was right in the midst of the main military build up by the Israeli's, on the Lebanese Border checkpoint on the main coastal route to Beirut, working in the Mitz Bar literally on the border crossing, a café/restaurant. I saw lots of soldiers from the United Nations and Israeli soldiers and the carrying of guns all over the place and tanks, it was a bit scary but exciting. After four months I left Israel, but not before back-packing around the Holy Land going to all the religious sights, which made an impact on me.

I went home to Loughton where I grew up. By this time my sister had left home to go to study physiotherapy at Middlesex University Hospital, so I was left with just my parents which was odd. I decided to move out to a flat, which I rented in Walthamstow in the East End of London. I was unemployed and felt a bit down and out, the action and adventure in Israel compared to living in a dingy flat in the East End really made me feel depressed. I joined an unemployment centre and made lots of friends there. I got really run down, had boils in my ears and went back home. My parents were abroad on a Far Eastern tour, so I recovered on my own. Shortly afterwards I got a job working as a forest surveyor for Epping Forest Conservation Centre. This was for about 6 months. I felt that it was strange living at home with my parents without my sister, and some of my friends had moved away.

The next thing I remember is my dad telling me that he was leaving home to 'be on his own'. After a couple of days we found out that he left the home to live with his girlfriend from his company that worked for him and not on his own as he had told us, this girl was married and the same age as me 21. I was furious and went hysterical, shortly afterwards her husband got her back and my dad was left on his own, apparently her husband went to my dad's work to beat him up.

About the time my dad told us he was leaving, there appeared on the front of the Loughton Gazette (local paper), a photo-fit picture of a man with the spitting image of my dad, when I saw this photo my blood ran cold and I almost fainted with fear, it was so like him, and the front page story ran like this – 'the police were looking for a man in connection with a serious assault and attempted rape (or rape) in Epping Forest'. I told my mother, and was convinced it was my dad, she said she didn't believe it was him and dismissed it. I later went to the theatre to watch Rowan Atkinson in a play with my sister and one of her friends with my dad, I was so nervous of him, and was waiting for a time when I could ask him if it was him that raped or attempted to rape this girl.

I waited until we were going to go in the auditorium and were gathered together in the bar area – I was so nervous and sweating but wanted to clear something up with my dad; I really don't know what I was doing there that evening with him, I was now petrified of him, I said 'dad, I saw this picture, which looked like you on the front of the Gazette of a man that raped or attempted to rape a girl' (I can't remember which it was now as it was so long ago) and I said 'was it you', and he just looked around and said 'of course it was me'. Well I was even more petrified that it was him and I couldn't sit still all through the evening at the theatre, even though it was Rowan Atkinson, I felt sweat pour down my face and couldn't wait to get out of there. This just went to reinforce what I felt about my alcoholic father. I was always scared of him. Some years later I was interviewed by two detectives about my concerns after I had met the police in the solicitors in London, I asked if I could clear this matter up, so consequently two detectives came and interviewed me from Epping to where I lived in Ilford, they took away a picture I had of my dad, and a copy of the newspaper article that Steve and I had traced back through Loughton library. When the police came back to me some time later, they told me that they got someone for the crime, some bloke called Godfrey and that he had confessed to doing this, but even now I wonder if it was a false confession that this bloke had made, I wouldn't put it past my alcoholic father in doing something like that, and why was he always so nasty to me, especially wanting me, later on to end up in 'chemical hand-cuffs' and to be 'silenced' with drugs.

Bye the way I should add that my dad was also a violent and aggressive and manipulative man; he had been physically violent to me on a number of occasions, punching me in the face, kicking me in the shins, slapping me violently around the head. He also rowed with my mother all the time and bullied her and was violent to her too, this went on for most of my teenage life, although he wasn't like this to my sister, mostly because I was the eldest and tried to protect my mother from him, as well as trying to break up the physical fights between my parents but all this was counteracted because we never went short for anything we needed and apart from my father everything was 'normal'?!

My mother was by this time working part time in a solicitors as a secretary, she had one of the female solicitors do the divorce for her (my mother now had the evidence she had wanted for years to get a divorce from him).

I decided to get a job working with horses in Wales; this was a plan of mine to leave my parents alone, because I thought if I'm not in the way they might get back together. (My dad told me that I had caused the breakup of their marriage), typical nasty thing my dad did and said, blame everyone else and never had any insight into himself; he still does this today, even though he doesn't drink alcohol anymore and hasn't done for a number of years he still is psychologically mixed up, blames everyone else, never says sorry for anything he has done to upset people and can never see that he ever does anything wrong, he has no guilty conscience at all, all the hallmarks of a psychopath.

Wales was a mistake, it rained all the time, I was totally upset by my parents marriage breakup, I couldn't talk to anyone there, I was bullied by some of the other stable girls who were from that area, and to add to that I sustained a really bad dislocated shoulder and had to return home.

That's when I started to become really depressed. I had to show prospective buyers around our family home, where we had two lovely cats and had a Labrador dog, it had been my home for five years and I had lived and been brought up in Loughton where I knew everyone, so many people, friends, teachers, shop workers, the whole fabric of my life was in Loughton and I knew nothing else. I can remember sitting in the hall of our home in Loughton after nearly everything had been cleared out, and sitting on the floor next to the front door, I just sat there my knees bent and head hanging down, saying to myself the 23rd Psalm 'even though I walk through the valley of the shadow of death I will fear no evil'.

My mother decided to live in Woodford Green, some 30 miles away from Loughton, near to her mother, my grandmother who lived there too. I had physiotherapy on my shoulder at Holly House private hospital, as I was still on the family's health insurance, which my dad took me off of shortly afterwards, another nasty thing he has done to me. (Later on I could have gone to a private hospital when I got into trouble but because my dad did this I had to suffer the consequences of a run-down NHS hospital with a history of abuse towards patients, as stories would often appear in the local paper). I even did some voluntary work there for a short time, but left in disgust and fear as to what was happening to the patients there, I was really upset by what I saw and could go into more detail about this too.

I went on holiday to the Greek Islands with one of my friends. I felt different now my parents were divorced, sort of lonely and alone. I was 22 and my friend had no idea of what I was going through, her parents were very happy together!

Some time later, I can't remember properly, about a year later I went back to the Greek Islands intending to find a suitable Greek man for a husband and live there forever away from England, my parent's bitter divorce, and bad weather. It was a good experience, but I ran out of money and had to come back to England after 6 months, but this was one of the best experiences of my life living on this remote Greek Island all on my own from May to September.

Came back to England, and then I had to live with my mother in a tiny little terraced house in

Woodford Green. (I have later found out that my mum settled for an out of court settlement in regards to the divorce as she didn't want the stress of coping with her ex husband who she was glad to see the back of, she only got half of what the house was worth and nothing more, so consequently my alcoholic father has been living off the sale of his business and pensions ever since in absolute luxury whilst my mother has suffered with living in a poor run down area of Ilford). I started going to Alanon meetings (this is the equivalent of Alcoholics Anonymous, for the wives, husbands, families and friends of alcoholics) with my mother, which I enjoyed, we got on o.k. at this time.

Because I had 'lost everything' which was dear to me, I was looking for answers, any answer that would make me feel better, because I felt so low, I contacted a clairvoyant, and went to a spiritualist church, I got scared and decided to go to the local Church of England to have a friendly talk to the vicar, who I thought would give me the comfort which I so badly needed. The vicar told me that I should 'go for prayer' with 'the people that pray over you'. So I started having prayer in the church after Sunday services and during the week when the 'Stepford Wives' (I later called them this because it was so strange looking back at it, the whole place was like 'The Crucible' as I was later to find out) could fit me in (in other words the rich middle class women that didn't work and had nothing better to do during the week than run prayer groups and bible studies), I was desperate for comfort, friends and help that could make me feel wanted and loved.

The prayer was weird, but powerfully intoxicating like a drug, it made me feel better – however, I started arguing with my mother at home. I kept telling her to go to church and she'll feel better like I was, and we constantly rowed. I was getting more and more 'brainwashed' by the whole bible, prayer and charismatic worship and got carried away to another planet. I then started praying all day, because I didn't have a job, and I had sold my horse and car to go travelling. So I prayed all day, did bible study all day, was totally cut off from 'normal every day' people because I only ever went to prayer groups and bible studies if there were any during the day and there was, and the relationship between me and my mother got worse. I belonged to 18+, a group of people my age. We went on holiday a couple of times together, they were more down to earth than a lot of the charismatic people at the other bible study groups and prayer groups. I also wanted to work in the church as a Deaconess or Evangelist but I wasn't encouraged enough.

This went on my about 5 years believe it or not. Until I got chucked out of the house by my mother, (she got the police to evict me, and guess what? The alcoholic father was behind a lot of it, he always did hate me anyway especially since the divorce) and then even worse things were to happen. (I was at this time about 29).

The events leading up to me being evicted by my mother were a bit confusing. Firstly about 6 or 7 months previously I went over to the police station in Woodford Green because I was concerned about what was going on, as far as I can remember it was because I didn't get on with my mother, I was completely brainwashed by what was happening to me at the church and I just wanted to get some 'reality' into my life, I wanted to leave home because my mother and me were at logger heads together and I was scared of her violent reactions to me, she had ignored me when I tried to talk to her about how I was feeling and I just felt a mess and I couldn't get out of the house; a few years previously when I came back from Greece I went to the local council in Ilford to try to get housing but they told me it was a five year waiting list and I naively thought 'I would be out of the house by then'. I even put an advertisement in the local parish newsletter asking if anyone had a room I could rent, but no-one responded – so much for Christian help! Looking back on it now, if only I had got out of that house my life would have been a whole lot different and all the bad things that happened to me probably would never occurred! I was also emotionally drained because of my parents divorce and the entire trauma that that had caused me.

My mother too, she has since told me that she was going through a hell of a lot because she had been married for 27 years and her getting divorced also had taken its toll on her. She worked full time as a legal secretary in London during this time, and I was on the dole, and no-one from the job centre ever tried to get me a job. (We have completely made up now and have been for some time, but at the time things were so painful). I had my dog who I loved, I had got him from the RSPCA in Nazing and enjoyed taking him for long walks through Epping Forest and round the golf course at Woodford Green. I was tired a lot during the day though. I tried to get 'more prayer', which was inadvertently me trying to talk to other people in the church about what I was going through, but some of the women who did the prayer were never available, and this just dragged on for months, they didn't want me to do any talking anyway they just wanted to 'pray over me', I had no-one to talk to about the terrible effects of my parents divorce the fact that my dad was an abusive violent alcoholic and had been for years and the loneliness

I felt in my life, the fact that we had moved to a new area, I had no friends in this area, a lot of my old friends from Loughton had moved away, and one of my old friends didn't want to know me anymore because I had become a 'born again' Christian. I had no car or horse anymore, I was poor, I didn't have any money or a job, all I had to cling on to was my faith and the church, my faith being the only thing I had and I knew that if I kept praying everything would be o.k. but this didn't happen at all and things got worse, but everyone at the church kept telling me it would get better – just keep praying they kept saying, as if prayer was the answer to everything but talking wasn't, and because I couldn't get prayer with these women a lot of the time I had to do all the praying on my own, I felt I was being palmed off by them as they couldn't offer any alternative to the prayer, this then led to me being victimised by them and 'framed up' when they told my mother, who I didn't get on with, that in their opinion 'there was something wrong with me', yes the only thing wrong with me was being gullible enough to go to the stupid church in the first place thinking that the church had all the solutions to life's problems and I was so naïve to think that people in the church were there to help, not in that church anyway, they probably knew that they couldn't do anything more for me, as they only thought that 'prayer' was the solution to all of life's problems. Because my mother and I didn't get on and we never communicated with each other, she listened to them at the church, and I was framed.

Looking back on this whole sordid story at this time I really needed counselling and a lot of it, probably two or three times a week, I needed to talk out everything that was going on. I was unable to talk about any of my problems to anyone in depth at that church and felt like I was just in a game of 'blind mans buff' where I was blindfolded and turned round and round by these church women and sent in all different directions. I had no-one to talk to, and I was getting confused. I have since found out a few years later, that a woman I had known at that church committed suicide, and another woman also had a nervous breakdown after going to that church.

It didn't occur to me to have counselling, I didn't even think about that at the time, I was too young and not knowledgeable about such things, my mind was totally focused on Jesus Christ being the only answer to my problems and the problems of everyone else, so I can relate to anyone who has experienced fundamentalist religion, I thought everyone in the world would be o.k. if they converted to Christianity, and I even said to myself that I would be a martyr for Jesus Christ, and turned my whole life over to His care not caring if I was killed for the sake of my faith.

I still loved my mother, despite all the difficulties we were having, and my grandmother who I used to visit across the golf course where she lived, and I loved living near the countryside of the forest where I used to spend a lot of time walking my dog Prince who was a Collie x Spaniel, and an unwanted dog who had had five homes before I rescued him from the animal sanctuary.

Anyway as I was saying I walked over to the police station one evening, and got talking to a police constable, I talked to him and he seemed quite friendly and took an interest in what I was saying. Some time later he came to visit me at home, his visits increased, and he asked me to go out with him for a drink. Bye the way he was a married man with 5 children, he was about the same age as me. But for me I never get involved with married men, and because I was a born again Christian I had decided not to get involved with any immorality. I thought he was just being friendly. Looking back on it now I realize that he had some other intentions. I was always a bit weary of him. We even prayed together – bizarre!

Some of the housewives who ran the bible study and prayer for people that needed it had ganged up on me, I began to question the prayer that they were giving and I told them that they weren't helping me, there was gossip in the church and it wasn't only me that they were prejudiced towards, they didn't like anyone that didn't fit the mould, which was coming from a 'normal' family, i.e. one that hadn't got divorced or anyone with problems for that matter, they were total hypocrites. It was becoming scary at the church, some people were not friendly towards me, especially some people of my age who were in the prayer groups, and I had been excluded from these prayer groups by one of the older women who didn't want me to join in with them, I rang her up and asked her why and she just said she didn't think I should be involved (she was also I think a teacher at a school). I was rejected and I felt so sad and rejected. I was so desperate for friends and in this prayer group were people of my own age. But also it had a sinister side in that a lot of them used to tell 'Satan to go away', all the time they were saying it in the group prayer, it scared me actually, but I wanted to be with some of the friends I had made.

Looking back on it now, the whole thing stinks to high heaven of making people like me outcasts from groups at the church, they really didn't care about me, none of them knew me, even though I had been to their prayer groups, they didn't ask about how I was coping with my parents divorce, the fact that I didn't know anyone in the area, or they didn't even know where I came from in Loughton and the life I lived beforehand, for some reason and I have found this at other churches, people in the church don't seem to want to know about your past, just what's going on in your life in relation to Jesus, and if you fit in with them, this is why I don't go to church now, because I have met more weirdo's in the church than anywhere else in the whole of my life, and I have met a lot of people that think the same way, although I still have my own personal faith and pray at times.

At some of these prayer groups they constantly talked about Satan, and constantly exorcised the whole thing by praying for Satan to go away. Even when I was receiving prayer, they didn't really know how bad I was feeling, all they did was a sort of exorcism on me telling Satan to go away and leave me alone, but the constant talk about Satan put a lot of fear into me, and I was already living in fear because I was insecure after my parents divorce, living in a new area, my dad had been round once and threatened to beat me up and I had to call the police, I was petrified of my dad, I was scared of my mothers violent reactions to me, she was always out at Alanon meetings, Alanon people rang her up all the time to talk to her about their alcoholic husbands and I felt utterly rejected by everybody. I knew either me or my mother were going to crack up because of the strain, and eventually it was me.

This particular policeman whose name will remain anonymous, took me out for a walk in Epping Forest, driving me there in his car when he was in his casual clothes not in uniform, and also asked me out for a drink one night in his car he drove me wearing his casual clothes. I tried to explain to him I needed to get of the house from living with my mother, I need some space – he totally ignored me. He did say he would go and visit the vicar to ask if there was anything he could do to help. I was also getting harassed by a woman in the church who got my phone number from somewhere and kept ringing me up and telling me I had to go round to her house for prayer. I had seen her and her husband on one occasion and felt really scared as they both practically pinned me to the sofa asking me how many boyfriends I had had in my life, they were weird, her husband Geoff worked as a youth worker in the church, they were both 'interrogating' me and I didn't like it, and didn't want to go there ever again, but this woman kept ringing me up, she wouldn't leave me alone.

Everything was getting out of hand. Somehow a curate from the church, who I noticed probably had a drink problem, somehow talked to my mother and said I needed to see a psychiatrist (I found this out later)…My mother told me one morning that a social worker would be coming round to see me. I thought that it was to help me leave home, and I wanted to speak to someone about leaving home ASAP. However, the person that turned up was a huge 6ft black man, driving a big Volvo car, and I was petrified. He came in, I think he introduced himself as a psychiatrist, and asked me some questions, one of which I can remember was 'am I a virgin'. I was so petrified by all of this, words cannot express how I felt, absolutely abandoned by everyone, and now they were all saying I was mad, and all I wanted to do was live in peace and be a Christian and leave home. I had at this time gone over to the Catholic Church and asked to be received there, as I had totally lost faith in the people at the Church of England, after what they had put me through, telling me that I needed more prayer, and I knew this wasn't the answer. After this black man had left, I flew into a rage, my mother was not in the room when this man was asking me all these questions, so when he had gone I went totally hysterical. I told my mother that she had betrayed me, she had lied to me, she told me that it was a social worker coming to see me, and I wanted to talk about leaving home. We argued and I was near to hysterics. (I locked her in the toilet... probably the worst mistake I have ever made, I was so annoyed at what she had done, and scared too of what she was planning behind my back). I then went to see the particular police constable to find out what the hell was going on to see if he had anything to do with the whole thing. I went to Woodford Green police station and he wasn't there, they told me that he was at Barkingside police station. So I took my dog and went over to Barkingside, where I couldn't find this particular PC. I went back to Woodford Green police station and walked calmly in there with my dog, a policeman asked me to sit down, I sat down with my dog next to me, all of a sudden about five burley policemen in uniforms came in grabbed me by my arms and started to physically pull me out of the room, they took my dog away from me. The violence of their action was destructive and scared me, and didn't even resist I was weak; I said to them 'you don't have to pull me; I'll go where you want me to go'. They bundled me into the back of a police van and drove madly away into the night, where I was going was anyone's business, but I was totally petrified and I thought they were taking me to a psychiatric hospital to have brain surgery.

I arrived at Barkingside police station where I watched a man being pushed onto the floor and handcuffed this was at the back of the police station where the cells were. I waited in this room and started to cry, I was really upset by what had happened and was totally scared and didn't know what was happening to me, my mother wasn't there nor was any of my family I felt all alone. After a while I was called into a room and a man in ordinary clothes came to talk to me with a PC watching, the PC that I knew turned up and hung around in the background. The man in the ordinary clothes asked me what was going on, I told him that 'I was a born again Christian and that my parents weren't and we didn't get on' (not to mention that my dad had a history of violence towards me). After that he went, and the PC that I knew came and asked me 'how much money I had on me', I said about £30.00, and with that he told me that they were going to take me to a place of safety. I was driven in a panda car to I didn't know where, but it turned out to be Ilford. I arrived at a house, went in with the woman PC and was left there. There was a big lounge with about 15 people in it sitting in relative darkness watching television. I was then shown to a room with a bed and bed clothes and nothing else, there were also a group of Asian men hanging around. At this time I was totally petrified of who these suspicious looking people were and the fact that I had to sleep in this place, a far cry from the relative safety of Woodford Green living in a quiet cul-de-sac with my mother, when my mother wasn't around I had peace anyway.

I think I prayed that night; I got the feeling that the next day I would follow this route that appeared to me when I prayed (probably though I knew from the past when travelling through Ilford that –

subconsciously there was a Catholic church there). The next morning I followed this route and ended up at a Catholic Church, I went to the presbytery and rang the bell and a nice looking priest answered the door I told him I needed to speak to him and he let me in to a comfortable room with table and chairs, I think he made me tea, and came back to talk to me. I poured out my heart to him, and he advised me to go and speak to the nuns who lived near by, he seemed to listen and care, but I was confused as to why I should then go and tell the whole story to the nuns as well. (In fact I did go and talk to one of the nuns, but they didn't seem to want to support me).

I can't remember when I went to speak to them but I went back to where I 'lived'. The rest is a nightmare of living at that place where the people that lived there had keys to my room and tried to scare me by opening my door in the night and sometimes I would find my bedclothes turned back, why? They knew I was helpless as I had been 'dumped' there by the police and had no recompense to them. There was only one cooker and about 30 people living in an eight roomed house, it was a total nightmare. Some of the younger residents watched horror videos at night, I was petrified. There was only one cooker, how were we all supposed to cook on that – 30 people?!! For breakfast I received a raw piece of streaky bacon and a raw egg – I suppose that's how they got away with calling themselves a 'bed and breakfast'?!

I managed to find out where the social security was, because I was in a new area, and had to register there for money to pay the landlord of this place. I was told that I would only have £20.00 a week to live on out of a maximum of £80.00 a week - £60.00 was to pay the Asian landlords that I saw.

Also on the first night that I 'arrived' at this place a social worker came and saw me, he seemed to care and asked me some questions like, 'are you alright' etc. Unfortunately for me he never turned up ever again so I never got the real help that I needed with my housing, even now I wonder why didn't he come back to check on me.

My cheques from the DSS were sent there and promptly went missing; obviously someone was stealing them there. I didn't receive any money for weeks, when I went to the local job centre to tell them they didn't want to know. I hardly had any money to live on and was relying on some money I had in the building society. I made arrangements for the cheques to be eventually picked up by me from the job centre to avoid them going missing, non of my family ever came to visit me, I phoned my dad in desperation but he was abusive and told me to go away, all my family had turned their backs on me, for one reason they didn't like me because I was a 'born again' Christian, I could go into this in more detail about my mother and sister how they didn't like me being a Christian, my dad didn't like it either, so the whole family turned against me.

I left this place after about 3 months only to go into another bed and breakfast which was nearly as bad as the first one, the people in these places were really weird, there was a so called child molester there and criminals, unmarried mothers a lot of immigrants who didn't speak English.

Because I couldn't do any hand washing in these places and a lot of my clothes needed washing I tried to go back home to ask my mother if I could do my hand washing there, but every time I went home she told me that I couldn't stay there otherwise she would call the police, she seemed very disturbed. I tried to talk to her but she didn't want to know.

When I was living in the second bed and breakfast my mind definitely began to flip, it was at night time when I was on my own, it was a nightmare situation and I couldn't get out of it, my mind couldn't cope with the destitution, shock, poverty, lack of food and squalor that I was living in, let alone the fact that everyone didn't want me anymore, not even the church, but I was not suicidal, I still felt somewhere deep inside that Jesus was looking after me.

One day after about 8 months I was round at my mothers and she called the police to take me away, because I didn't want to go back to living in hell in a squalid room, I wanted her to help me get out of the situation I was in. Anyway the police came and took me to Barkingside police station and put me in a cell. I was there for quite a while, sat quietly and waited. I was then taken to Claybury Psychiatric hospital. I had worked there as a volunteer for a while when I was about 23 and thought the place was like purgatory, and left shortly afterwards after seeing terrible abuse of patients there.

I was at this hospital for two weeks minding my own business thinking that someone would come and help me sort my housing problem out, and I actually felt a sort of happiness because I was with people and thought that they cared about my housing situation. (I didn't have any psychosis at this time, the only time I felt my brain couldn't cope was when I was alone at night), when one evening I was told by a male nurse that if I didn't take the pill he was holding then I would be forced to take it. I saw an old lady being forced to have an injection a few days before when they had her on the floor, it was disgusting to witness, and looking back on it now I realise that she probably had senile dementia. As God is my witness for the two weeks I was there waiting for a solution to my housing situation I was as calm as a cucumber, if only I had known that I was free to leave whenever I wanted to, I was not on a 'section' at that time and totally oblivious to the psychiatric system and everything official and 'one's rights'.

Obviously things were talked about behind my back, without my knowledge, as I had never even talked to any doctor about why I had ended up there and what was the cause of me ending up there. Obviously my parents, especially my alcoholic father, had filled the doctors in on what they deemed my 'inappropriate behaviour', namely just being a brainwashed born again Christian, I prayed and I knew that my dad was behind a lot of this, he had turned my mother against me once again, and I was scape-goated once again, (he seemed to have got even worse towards me since the divorce).

One night I was on my own in the corridor of the ward and a male nurse came up to me with a couple of pink pills in his hand, he said 'that if I didn't take these pills I would be forced to against my will', I remembered the old lady squashed on the floor with several nurses on top of her forcing her to have an injection, and thought that I could die if I was in that situation, and so I thought of a passage in the bible where it said something like 'even though you take poison, it will not harm you'. So I inevitably took the pink pill that fateful night and things were never the same again. I then turned into a drugged up zombie and became a shadow of my former self, I couldn't keep my eyes open during the day and kept falling asleep all the time.

The most horrifying thing was happening to me, I would get terrible distortions of my body and my neck would twist round so that I thought my neck was going to snap it practically turned round 90 degrees, but nobody did anything about it, also my eyes would go right round in their sockets so that I couldn't see anything, and when my parents came to see me, do you know what my dad said to me 'You're doing that on purpose so that you don't get any more drugs' my mother was with him but didn't do anything. Then shortly afterwards when this was happening again two nurses took me into a side room and questioned me, they were laughing at me and telling me not to be stupid. I can't remember their names, but I can only describe them as totally evil. They kept me on this drug for six months, in which time my hair fell out, I couldn't brush my teeth because I couldn't hold my toothbrush properly and I definitely couldn't communicate properly because I was drugged up with the drug from hell.

Even the curate from my old church turned up but he wasn't even coming to see me, but someone else he knew at the hospital. No one from my old church came to see me, I hardly had any visitors, my parents hardly came and saw me.

During this time on this ward there was mayhem, a boy committed suicide or someone set him alight I never found out, he died. I was talking to him the day previously or trying to talk to him through the haze of drugs, and then he was dead. No staff on that ward cared. There was no permanent doctor there only locums that kept coming and going it was total mayhem. I told a member of staff that I felt suicidal, nothing was done about it. The only reason I felt like killing myself was because I was suffering pain being on the drugs they kept forcing me to take every day, every day I had to line up for a drug that was making me ill and no one did anything about it, if you refused to take them you would be forced to have an injection into the buttocks with a group of nurses sitting on you, like I had already witnessed. Also I was nearly raped whilst trying to walk in the grounds, when a male black man tried to get me to walk with him into the forest, but because I was so drugged up I couldn't protect myself, and was lucky to escape from him.

I got to a train station on one occasion after trying to escape from that hell of a place. I had walked to Epping Forest from where the hospital was and walked to a pond where I met a man that was fishing, I had told him I had run away from the hospital and he told me that he had been in prison, I told him that I was being forced to take pills against my will and that they were making me ill, I could hardly talk because the drug that I was on, being haloperidol, had seized up my throat, he told me that in prison he had had the 'liquid cosh' himself, I was telling him all this when my neck, on its own accord, starting turning round and round till I thought my neck was going to snap I couldn't control it, I couldn't look forwards and was looking over my shoulder. This man said he would take me to a train station when his lift turned up. Anyway I was dropped off at Chingford train station, moving my limbs around helped with the contortions, and I boarded a train to Liverpool Street station. It was so embarrassing on the train, my neck was craning sideways and now my body was twisting out of control my arms were twisting round, I must have looked like a deformed monster, and I was wondering what people were thinking. Anyway I got to my

destination and then I thought I would get on a train and head for the Catholic Church and go and see the priest I knew, namely Father Sheil. I got to Goodmayes station in Ilford near to where the church was, by this time it was dark and I found myself staring at the train track, I was out of it, and really I had no-one to turn to, I don't even know if Father Sheil was going to help. I stood there on the side of the train track trying to fathom out which part of the station would be best for putting myself in front of the train and not causing a mess, I just wanted to get rid of the excruciating pain in my body that I was feeling being on this drug, I couldn't decide, so I left the station and went to see the priest I knew, I was totally out of it because of this weird drug. I met Father Sheil in the church where he was with some other parishioners, they all seemed concerned, I couldn't talk and practically collapsed in front of them, I was taken to the presbytery where I passed out. The next thing I knew I was being driven back to the hospital from hell, where a night nurse greeted me calmly, the night staff always were a lot kinder than the day staff.

I left after 6 months of sheer hell and nothing had improved I was still told I had to take these pink horrible pills that made me into a numb, senseless zombie with a stiff wooden body and I couldn't talk properly to explain how I felt, the drug had paralyzed me all over my body including my voice box and throat. I can't begin to describe how I felt on these drugs – I felt worthless and a victim – a powerless victim, I couldn't communicate properly which only made things worse, because this drug had seized up my throat.

I now found that I only had one place to live other than the hospital was a half way house or hostel run by the local council – another den of iniquity, which I found myself in after being discharged from hospital.

In this place there were all sorts of people with mental health problems, there was a boy with some sort of brain damage, and generally people seemed really out of it, they were all men too, they walked around aimlessly from one room to another in there own mental hell. I made friends with a man called Mike who was there for depression; he was about the only 'normal' person there that I could have a decent conversation with. We used to go to the pub down the road, also with a chap named Andrew who was a bit chaotic. There I was a drugged up shadow of my former self, when I looked back at how I was before my parents got divorced and everything I had, now I was living in a social services hostel with no money and hardly anything to my name, only the clothes I stood up in.

I decided to come off the drugs myself as they were making me so ill, and I immediately felt better. However, after six months of having a good time things got slightly out of hand. I had during this time gone back to the Catholic Church where I had made such good friends with the priest there, and was taking classes to become a catholic. I used to walk about 5 miles every evening to go to evening mass at this church. However I was rarely visited by my parents and never saw my sister at all, I think in the last 15 years since she had left home I could count the times I had seen her on one hand.

One of the staff assaulted me and I retaliated, he then tried to break my arms and I screamed. I got the police involved, they didn't want to do anything. Other illegal things were going on in this hostel that I don't think I have the time to write at this moment.

Because I had caused trouble I ended up being taken to hospital again. I was put in a locked ward and because I didn't want to take the pink pills that made me so ill, I was then forced to have injections in the backside being jumped on one afternoon by a group of nurses – I'm sure that they got some sick sense of satisfaction out of doing this kind of thing. I had no choice I never had the opportunity of talking to a doctor or consultant about anything. The locked ward was yet another place of hell, I saw an old man punched in the face by one of the male nurses, and I was forced to do the sweeping of the eating area and do the washing and wiping up, it was on a rota. I was so drugged up I didn't know what I was doing, I didn't have a lot of energy and pushing a broom around was an effort, everything was an effort, the drugs this time were not causing physical pain in my body but making me so lethargic that I could hardly move. (I could go into more detail about the horrors that went on there including what happened to me, thankfully this hospital was closed in the mid to late 90's, what is scary though is what happened to all the abusive staff? Where did they all go to?).

Sometimes looking back at all this I question the fact 'was it all necessary'? It all seems such a waste of a life, and if anyone with any intelligence was looking into this they may have rescued me from the hell that I was going through. I even went to a tribunal to appeal to get out of there but was turned down, I was so drugged up that I could hardly make sense of what I was saying, and to think that in the past women and men like me would have been forced to have operations on their brains instead of the pink horrible pills. And I used to read in the local Loughton Guardian of brutality by nurses at this hospital and now I was witnessing it myself and it was happening to me.

Was all this necessary, no wonder I later got depressed after having a great deal of my life wasted because when it comes down to it 'nobody really cared about me'.

After being at this hospital again for about 2 months I was released and went back to the half way hostel to hell. It was not long afterwards that I moved into my own flat, a studio flat that measured 12ft x 14ft a box room to live in, but at least it was my own space and I felt grateful that for all the years I had tried to get away from living with my mother I had at last got somewhere to call my own home – (bit of a long way round to getting your own housing though isn't it?!) What a waste of time the whole episode was. However, I was heavily medicated still, but having to have injections. I ballooned to about 5 stone heavier than I should be. I went to a slimming club, got down to a proper level and soon met a nice boyfriend called Steve. We went out with each other for ages, he was a very good friend of mine and a good listener, and we still keep in touch today.

During all this time of all this hell happening to me, my parents had got back together, not as husband and wife, but as business partners (my mother says now that it was the worst decision she has ever made, I also found out later that they were seeing each other when I first became a born again Christian). They had started up their own business together selling books imported from American. My dad had bought the business from someone. Looking back now I remember before all this happened to me when I was still living in Woodford Green, my grandmother telling me that my parents were going into business together and we both knew this spelt disaster, I should have realized then that my mother getting back with my dad in any way was bad, especially for me because my dad hated me and this influenced my mother, especially as we didn't get on as I was religious and she wasn't. I can remember my nan and me talking about it even then and saying it was a mistake for them to do this, even my nan knew the capabilities of my dad, but whilst they were married and we all lived together my dad couldn't get to me because my mother protected me, but after they got divorced,....well it all went completely wrong.

However, my mother seemed quite happy now that I was drugged up and not going to church, and suggested that I work part time at their business, so she came and picked me up from Woodford Green to Ilford and then drove to Waltham Abbey, where I was so tired due to the drugs that I couldn't keep my eyes open and couldn't do any work at all, but I got some cash in hand for doing nothing. I used to go to my mother's car during the day and sleep in it, sitting there just slumped in a stooper a drugged up, fat and ugly looking girl, such a long way from where I originally came from, with parties, disco's, boyfriends, job, travelling abroad, a horse etc., etc.

Anyway I confided in Steve about all that had happened to me and he seemed really caring and we had some good times together. We went to Italy to visit his step father and used to go out with my friend Mike from the half way house (he had now moved to Stratford) with Mike's friends etc. The injections I was on were gradually reduced; I always kept insisting that they be reduced so that I didn't feel so drugged up and tired. Some days I couldn't get out of bed because the drugs made me so tired, I would sleep until 3 p.m. sometimes.

The consultant I was seeing said to me on a couple of occasions that he didn't think that the drugs were necessary because I was on such a low dose that in his opinion 'they weren't having any effect' and that I could safely come off of them. I felt great, this was great news that I was cured and didn't need to go on any more drugs of any sort. I can remember now that every time the drugs were reduced I would go out and celebrate. Most of the time in the beginning I couldn't work because the drugs made me so tired, but over a couple of years things began to improve and I did a word processing course, passed exams and did a work placement for a year in a government job club. I wasn't paid though, I was now about 34. I tried desperately to get a paid job at this time, filling in loads of application forms and going to interviews, but I wasn't 'lucky' enough to get a paid job, because of the recession it was difficult.

When I came off the drugs I was so happy. I used to see my Nan all the time. The relationship between my mother and I had improved. About this time, my parents business went bankrupt and my mother nearly lost her house in Woodford Green, it was nearly repossessed in the recession under the Conservatives in the mid – late 90's. My mother lost about £30,000. She had to move and bought a one bed roomed ground floor flat in a poor and run down part of Ilford, moving just down the road to where I actually lived. (Getting involved with my dad was always doomed to disaster) – Notably my dad wasn't affected he still lived in a period terraced cottage in a very posh part of Loughton next to Epping Forest, (Does anyone or can anyone really see what this man has done?) My mother also began to tell me about the abuse she suffered whilst working with my dad, in that he would physically become violent towards her, and one time tried to spray furniture polish in her eyes. Nowadays she has nothing to do with him.

I started getting on very well with my mother, especially when she wasn't influenced by Mr. Parsons, (this is what we call him).

I was now about 36 and decided to try to look into the whole mess that I got into. I started by going to my MP in Ilford, Mike Gapes a Labour Party MP, who advised me to go through the Police Complaints Authority about the initial problems with the PC and where I ended up, in that it was not a place of safety and made my health get worse, also a social worker had been appointed to me when I first went into the B & B but I only saw him once, he never kept in touch. I tried to get a solicitor to help me but a lot of them didn't want to handle the case, I don't know why, it probably seemed too complicated I was ringing a lot of them up and having to go over the whole story on the phone, (thank God for computers and emailing these days!) Also I wasn't well informed about which solicitor could handle police negligence and medical negligence and hardly any solicitors wanted to help with the police complaint. Although I did get someone and eventually met some police from the internal affairs in the solicitor's office in London, although this solicitor eventually didn't want to proceed with the case, I was upset. I kept ringing round solicitors and trying to tell my story but it was so long and complicated and I was getting anxious again, I was reliving the whole thing day and night, I had to write out statements for the police and solicitors and it went on and on and I got into a mess with the whole thing. I broke up with Steve and had to do it all on my own. I didn't get any support from my mother, she didn't think what I was doing was a good thing. I never saw my dad and didn't even want to. And as for my sister, as usual she was non existent as ever, and never helped at all. (I did in fact get a solicitor in the end but because of what happened next I was pressurized into not progressing with the case by my then GP).

In the end I had another breakdown and ended up in hospital in Goodmayes when I was about 38. I asked to take the drugs myself, I remember someone telling me years ago that if I ever ended up in hospital again to ask for Melleril which was a sedating drug with hardly any side effects, so I went in voluntarily to hospital as I knew I needed help and asked for this drug, they gave this to me (I had by this time been 4 years drug free). I was taking this drug for about a week, when unexpectantly one evening I was told I was to take another pill, I did this and WHAM... it was the same again as the haloperidol the pink pill, my head craned up to the ceiling on its own accord, my body became stiff all over like a sort of riga mortis, I couldn't talk my throat had seized up, just like the haloperidol I had been forced to take years ago, I managed with some effort to shuffle really slowly, every movement was so painful to the door of the dormitory and then into the corridor, I tried to look left and right to see who was there but I couldn't turn my head round without extreme pain,

I couldn't talk, there was a woman standing next to me looking out the window, she began talking to me but I couldn't answer her, I saw one of the male nurses walk past and wanted to tell him that this drug was making me ill, he was rushing about, eventually he stopped because I was standing stock still in the corridor and I managed to squeak out something to him, but he just ignored me and walked away. (I would like to point out at this point I had not talked to a doctor about anything, I was a voluntary patient, and had not discussed my treatment with anyone).

The next day I was told I had to go to a meeting. I turned up at the room appointed, inside were about five or six men, some with white coats on. I was asked to sit down, I sat. I was told that the drug I was taking (which was making me physically and mentally ill) was going to be given to me in injection form. Well, I just felt my stomach plummet to the floor and the blood drain out of my face, 'are you sure'? I thought. I still couldn't communicate properly or if at all, I just walked out of the meeting in total shock. (I remembered overhearing my alcoholic father outside a door telling someone that 'I was better when I was on injections', and that's how he always managed to get one over on me, especially when I was an over-weight drugged up nothing of a person. He had been telling people this and other lies in the hospital, when I was quite willing to take the drugs myself, so long as they weren't making me ill. I walked around for a while trying to think what I was going to do, and all I came up with was 'leave the hospital, go, run away', so I left. I think at this time I saw an advocate in the hospital and had a telephone number of a solicitor.

I left the hospital, walked to where I lived, knocked on a neighbour's door, and went in to talk to my Irish neighbours Anne and Willie who I had often gone and had a cup of tea with. I asked Willie if he could go and get me a few items of clothes namely warm ones from my flat, as I didn't want to go there incase I would be seen. He came back with a few items (I had told them what had happened to me). I went and left to go to Stratford to Mike's house. I got there only to find that Mike had died three weeks earlier, and funny enough I got this feeling a few weeks earlier that I had to contact Mike. I was too late. I stayed the night at his dwellings with his friend Alan and another flat mate. I remember going for a walk and crossing the road, weirdly enough my mother was just going down the road with her friend Joe in the passenger seat, right I thought she'll know where I'm staying. I decided to leave Alan's and headed for London. I ended up sleeping rough outside Victoria Station with some backpackers. I rang emergency housing phone lines for the homeless, and found somewhere at Shepherds Bush. I went there, stayed there for about three weeks. I knew I would be found sooner or later. I was found eventually and taken back to Goodmayes. It was night time, I felt 'happy' to be back because I knew something had changed, when I turned up I was put in another part of the building (I later found out that my mother had gone mad when she found out that I had walked out, and had gone to the Chief Executives office in the main hospital building and practically kicked the door down).

I was in Pathways, the intensive unit of the hospital, where inadvertently Frank Bruno was some years later. I was given some liquid to swallow, I drank it, and I didn't feel too bad. The next day I didn't have any painful bodily extortions and could communicate. Everyone in this ward was really o.k. and I felt sort of 'at home' there, there was a relaxed feeling, even the food there was better. A young doctor, a woman, came and talked to me whilst I was sitting down, and asked me what had happened, this was a change! We talked about drugs, what was the best one for me, as I had told her about why I walked out of the hospital; I said I would have no problem with taking the drugs myself. This was agreed and I was then put on a small amount of this drug, even one of the other patients complained loudly that I was only taking a small amount compared with him when we all lined up at night to take our 'medicine'. I got a solicitor who got me out of there in no time at all. That was all 8 years ago. I was impressed by the professionalism in this unit and thanked them all for their help, and sent everyone, all the patients a Christmas card when I got out and sent the staff a card of thanks for their help; I had never been treated so well in any hospital admission before.

I gradually got the drug I was on reduced to practically the lowest amount possible and now only take a tiny little bit every night to ensure that I go to sleep and who wouldn't need to get help getting to sleep after everything I have been through.

A few weeks after leaving hospital I was talking to my advocate that I had in hospital and she told me that she took anti-depressants and they really helped her, I was telling her I was feeling a bit low, quite low in fact. We went together to an out-patient appointment, and I was prescribed anti-depressants, and have been on them now for 8 years gradually having them increased because I asked for them to be increased, as I would cry and feel terribly upset by all the losses I had felt and gone through. My diagnosis is now Depression, that's what my friendly GP told me, and I'm not surprised I got depressed after everything that has happened to me. I feel that I have lost out on a career and the prospect of having children and marriage, but I try not to think of that too much, at least I can do something about my career, and if anyone nice does come along that'll be o.k. I try to keep focused on the future and the good things that I can do, and focus also on the present, living here and now, not looking back because the past is just a memory and you can't change the past. I feel that I am doing o.k. on these anti-depressants and at present don't want to come off of them as I feel that they really help.

I did get back with Steve for two years, but he didn't want to move in with me, and wanted to stay living with his mother. (By this time I had got a transfer to a housing association flat, which was a lot bigger and a lot better in another part of Ilford.) Anyway I felt he was too immature for me and I had moved on and been through a lot and he didn't seem to want to be there for me, as I found out he had had other relationships when we broke up, things were just not the same.

My grandmother died 10 years ago, and my grandfather on my dad's side, whom I also loved, died about 9 years ago. I miss them both. I always thought I would love to see more of my grandfather but I couldn't risk seeing my alcoholic father at the old people's home where he lived for the last six years after moving from the South coast.

The alcoholic father lives in relative luxury in a four bed roomed house in Hertfordshire, where he was living with his girlfriend of 11 years whom he met in Alcoholics Anonymous, she was 15 years his junior, he recently married her and they were married for two years, she has since left him and he has just gone through his second divorce, he had to pay her £80,000 in the divorce settlement, whilst I have hardly received a penny from him in 23 years since his first divorce. I don't have anything to do with him, he hasn't worked for years but lives off all the money he had retained after the divorce, has a gardener and a cleaner working for him and is a totally self-centred, spiteful and resentful man.

In the last 8 years I have done a great deal. I usually go on holiday with my mother to Spain every year. I had two cats, both rescue cats from charities, although one of them, Coco a Persian, died about six weeks ago but I have made plans to get an Exotic kitten (half Persian x British

Shorthair). My mother has tried to make up for a lot of the bad things that have happened to me, she helps pay my bills (which I hate) but have no choice when I am living on Incapacity Benefit which is below the so called bread line, being under £100.00 per week for everything in life's needs, including utility bills. I am stuck in the 'benefits trap'. I have been trying to gain qualifications in which to work, and have worked some of the time, as an audio typist in an accountants, and in an animal sanctuary, and as gym instructor, and with young offenders, I even passed a telephone interview and had my c.v. accepted for a job in MI5, which I still have the documents that prove that this happened, I still could go into this further but feel that because I have had a bit of a roller-coaster life I'm not sure how this would all fit in, if at all.

These are the exams and qualifications I have gained over the last 8 years;

1. Direct Computer Training (Ilford) City & Guilds NVQ Level 3 Information Technologies (Word, Excel, and PowerPoint 2001)

2. YMCA Gym Instructor Award NVQ Level 2 2002.

3. IIHH Body Massage Certificate NVQ Level 3 2002.

4. YMCA Nutrition NVQ Level 3 2002

5. Jobwise College (London) Diploma (Distinction) for Reception/Switchboard Duties (Monarch 120, Meridian and ISDX consoles) 2004.

6. Information Horizons Dreamweaver MX Certificate (website design) 2005.

7. Counselling & Psychotherapy Central Awarding Body Certificate for Initial Counselling Skills 2005.

My other qualifications before this time were as follows;

3 O'Levels: Art, English Language, Secretarial Duties.

1 R.S.A. Typing I.

4 C.S.E.'S. Social Studies, Typing, Biology, Shorthand.
(All 1977 and 1978.) Did 1 year of History of Art A'Level in sixth form.

GPO trained PABX 1 10 X 30 switchboard 1979.
Sight & Sound College (London) 100 w.p.m. shorthand 1981.
Weatherby Examination Services Diploma's WordPerfect 5.1 Basic, and WordPerfect 5.1 Advanced Word Processing. 1993.
Audio and Copy Typing speed 60+ w.p.m.

I also have a clean and current driving license. I have been on Jury Service twice in the last eight years, once at a lengthy case at the Old Bailey. I have had no criminal convictions in my life and have had an enhanced CRB check with nothing on it.

I am currently completing a correspondence course in Life Coaching. This September I am due to start about six new courses which are, Counselling Theory and Skills Certificate (with a friend of mine, which is one step away from a Counselling Diploma, which I hope to do the following year), Sculpture and Clay Modeling, another course in Website Design, Yoga (with a view to teaching Yoga in the future), Abstract Art at the City Lit near Covent Garden, and maybe Swimming Coaching. I'm just keeping all my options open.

I belong to two social organizations and have done a lot with them over the last few years and have hosted some events especially at over 35's nightclubs and have been out and about quite a lot. I got a new car a year ago, a Volkswagen Polo, previous to that I had my mum's old car a Fiat Panda, and I have, so far, in my life never been involved in a car accident or had any driving points against me!! I belong to the Ramblers Association and have done a lot of long distance walks, at one time I was going to the gym about 4 or 5 times a week for a couple of hours and doing 15 mile walks at the weekend, sometimes Saturday and Sunday, I was very fit, and still keep myself fit.

I don't get involved with the church anymore as I see a lot of the people there as hypocrites and gossipers. (Too many bad experiences with these types of people), I did keep in touch with some nuns I knew but they have moved away from the area, one of them died and the other one is in her 90's, I speak to her by phone sometimes. I do still have my own personal faith and do pray sometimes which I find beneficial. I also meditate and try to keep my life on an even keel.

My mother still works, despite being over retirement age, full time as a counsellor and has been doing this for about 10 years, she works as a counsellor to the relatives of alcoholics, which could be partners, parents or children of alcoholics as they need just as much support living with someone with a drink related problem as anyone else, as my life has shown. I don't have much to live on with Incapacity Benefit and if it wasn't for my mother helping me then I wouldn't be doing half the things that I am doing now. I have written to my MP Mike Gapes in the Labour Party about the fact that I live below the poverty line, but he just sends my letters to another department and I get a standard reply from them.

My dad never helped me at all. All the time I was living in poverty after I left hospital and went into my first flat. He used to send me postcards from other countries abroad where he was on holiday with his 'lady friend'. I used to walk around in second hand clothes and shoes I was so poor.

What I'm trying to say is all of this over the last 17 years need not happened all those years ago if I could get appropriate housing, as there was about five year waiting list with the council then I couldn't get out of Woodford Green, and private landlords wouldn't take DSS money, so I gradually got more and more stuck and more and more dependant on that stupid church, when all I needed looking back now was someone normal to talk to about my parents splitting up like a counsellor and somewhere else to live.

I now live in rented accommodation at the age of 45, I have missed out on a career, and have missed out on finding a suitable partner and having a family of my own, something I wanted a great deal earlier on in my life as I come from a very small family. The only members of my family that are left are just my mother and sister, not counting my alcoholic father, because my parents were both only children I have no uncles and aunts or near cousins, but have some relatives on my dads side which he doesn't like me getting involved with.

The Incapacity Benefit I live on is only £92.00 a week and out of that I'm supposed to pay all my bills – gas, water, electricity, phone etc., not to mention my weekly living expenses and household expenses. My dad never helps me out with money, however my mother does. I know it's not good to be reliant on anyone else to pay my bills but it's either this or die of starvation, lack of heating and electricity, no phone or internet etc. It's a shame that the government can't see that helping people like me with a good education etc. might pay off in the long run, I would like to be self-employed, but all this is in the pipe-line.

I know my local MP quite well as I have been quite an active member of the Labour Party for the past 11 years and I know him socially so he knows, to a certain extent what I have been through, although I know that my alcoholic father has been to see him, and I'm sure he's put in a bad word about me.

A lot of ex-addicts have personality disorders so this is very hard to cope with, my dad is also a compulsive liar and totally does my brain in, for example he is not a qualified counsellor, but I noticed on his business card when I last visited him that he says on his business card that he has a diploma in counselling, this is a three year course, and I know for a fact that he has only done an introduction to counselling course a number of years ago, this is only one of many lies that he tells, he also doesn't care who he lies to, I think he does it to impress people but what's the point? Does he feel so inadequate about himself? One day I might fathom out exactly what makes my dad 'tick'.

Also I have met a lot of prospective boyfriends over the last eight years, I have had quite a lot of dates, but mainly I find a lot of the men have 'gone off the rails', and are into addictions, like sex addiction (trying to get me to go to a swingers club), having a number of girlfriends at the same time like one for every day of the week, some have been weird, one was a compulsive gambler and liar, another had a terrible food problem and drink problem he also had a long criminal record. I have actually met 18 different men or even more and not one of them has been suitable, not at all kind enough or anywhere near intelligent, I think it is the area I am living in. I am quiet attractive and still value my own self worth despite what I have been through, I am tall, have blonde hair and green eyes and slim and keep myself fit, some people have said that I could be a model. I have had professional photo's done of myself and sometimes use them on internet dating sites, but no-one intelligent enough has ever come my way yet!

What do I think after everything that has happened to me? Well, I only found out four months ago that I'm being treated for depression, my GP told me whom I am on quiet friendly terms with, he showed me what was written about me on his computer screen, then this leads to the question – then what was all the past 17 years been about, if

I was depressed when all this first happened and am depressed now (or at least taking anti-depressants for depression), then what was everything that occurred in between?! Is it right to deal with people like I have been dealt with?? I also have no pension for my future and have to rebuild my career from scratch, so at present I am also looking once again at a possible legal case, because I was told some years ago that I was a schizophrenic by one or two nasty doctors who seem to get some sick satisfaction out of saying those words, and these were spoken when I was on my own and when the doctor seemed to be in quite a mood, and I never have believed it neither has my mother, who is now staunchly on my side and will help me in a legal case, this is what she says. For some years now there has been a lot of shuffling around with different consultants and doctors with differing opinions, and they seem to by-pass the question of 'what the Label is'? There has definitely been a shift away from what was originally said, and I really can't believe that that was ever the case, but I know I was suffering from a stress related illness, either anxiety due to events or depression due to events and this is what I want to prove in a legal case if I can get anyone to represent me.

This is where I am currently at in my life.

August 2006

www.ingramcontent.com/pod-product-compliance
Lightning Source LLC
Chambersburg PA
CBHW031931080426
42734CB00007B/631